Mediterranean Dash Diet Simple & Delicious Recipes

A Set of Quick and Easy Recipes for Your Mediterranean Dash Diet Meals

Kathyrn Solano

© **Copyright 2021 - All rights reserved.**

The content contained within this book may not be reproduced, duplicated or transmitted without direct written permission from the author or the publisher.

Under no circumstances will any blame or legal responsibility be held against the publisher, or author, for any damages, reparation, or monetary loss due to the information contained within this book. Either directly or indirectly.

Legal Notice:

This book is copyright protected. This book is only for personal use. You cannot amend, distribute, sell, use, quote or paraphrase any part, or the content within this book, without the consent of the author or publisher.

Disclaimer Notice:

Please note the information contained within this document is for educational and entertainment purposes only. All effort has been executed to present accurate, up to date, and reliable, complete information. No warranties of any kind are declared or implied. Readers acknowledge that the author is not engaging in the rendering of legal, financial, medical or professional advice. The content within this book has been derived from various sources. Please consult a licensed professional before attempting any techniques outlined in this book.

By reading this document, the reader agrees that under no circumstances is the author responsible for any losses, direct or indirect, which are incurred as a result of the use of information contained within this document, including, but not limited to, — errors, omissions, or inaccuracies.

Table of contents

GREAT MEDITERRANEAN DIET RECIPES 6
- White Bean Veggie Burgers 6
- Chicken N' Orange Salad Sandwich 8
- Avocado toast 9
- Overnight Oats 10
- Cabbage slaw 12
- Roasted grape crostini with ricotta and balsamic reduction 13
- Low sodium herbed grilled corn 15
- Sour candy Grapes 16
- Incredible raspberry pear sorbet 17
- Cherry brown butter bars 18
- Honey garlic kebab marinade 20
- Grilled blackened tilapia 21
- Zucchini and Feta Cake 22
- Steamed Vegetables served with Macadamia Dressing 24
- Broccoli a la Polonaise 26
- Broccoli, cauliflower & feta salad 27
- Lentils, Zucchini & Tomato Sauce 28
- Pumpkin with Butternut Curry 29
- Simple Sautéed Cauliflower 31

BREAKFAST & LUNCH 33
- Egg, Prosciutto, And Cheese Freezer Sandwiches 33
- Veggie Mediterranean Quiche 35
- Mediterranean Scrambled Eggs 38
- Chia Pudding 40
- Breakfast Rice Bowls 41
- Tahini Egg Salad With Pita 42
- Strawberry-mango Green Smoothie 44
- Breakfast Taco Scramble 45
- Whole-wheat Pancakes With Spiced Peach And Orange Compote 47
- Peanut Butter Banana Greek Yogurt 49
- Green Shakshuka 50
- Clean Breakfast Cookies 52
- Omelet With Cheese And Broccoli 54
- Greek Yogurt Breakfast Bowl 56
- Cucumber Celery Lime Smoothie 57
- Chocolate-almond Banana Bread 58

MEDITERRANEAN BREAKFAST EGG WHITE SANDWICH	60
STRAWBERRY-APRICOT SMOOTHIE	62
APPLE QUINOA BREAKFAST BARS	63
PEPPER, KALE, AND CHICKPEA SHAKSHUKA	65
ROSEMARY BROCCOLI CAULIFLOWER MASH	67
PUMPKIN, APPLE, AND GREEK YOGURT MUFFINS	68
BACON BRIE OMELET WITH RADISH SALAD	71
CRANBERRY OATMEAL	73
RICOTTA FIG TOAST	74
MUSHROOM GOAT CHEESE FRITTATA	75
HONEY, DRIED APRICOT, AND PISTACHIO YOGURT PARFAIT	77
MEDITERRANEAN STUFFED SWEET POTATOES WITH CHICKPEAS AND AVOCADO TAHINI	78
WALNUT BANANA OATMEAL	81
SUPER-SEED GRANOLA	82
HAM AND EGG MUFFINS	84
ALMOND PANCAKES	86
MEDITERRANEAN EGG MUFFINS WITH HAM	88
OVERNIGHT BERRY CHIA OATS	90
QUINOA	91
EGG, FETA, SPINACH, AND ARTICHOKE FREEZER BREAKFAST BURRITOS	92
LOW CARB WAFFLES	94
POTATO BREAKFAST HASH	95
FARRO PORRIDGE WITH BLACKBERRY COMPOTE	96
BULGUR FRUIT BREAKFAST BOWL	98
ACORN SQUASH EGGS	100
GREEN SMOOTHIE	102
THICK POMEGRANATE CHERRY SMOOTHIE	103
HONEY NUT GRANOLA	104
QUINOA GRANOLA	106
GREEK YOGURT WITH FRESH BERRIES, HONEY AND NUTS	108

GREAT MEDITERRANEAN DIET RECIPES

White Bean Veggie Burgers

Preparation time: 10 minutes
Cooking time: 15 minutes
Servings:

Ingredients:

1 cup white beans
1 cup White rice cooked
1 tsp Garlic powder
2 tsp dried thyme
½ tsp Ground chipotle pepper
½ chopped sweet onion
½ cup of corn
½ cup chopped red bell pepper
2 tbsp Lemon Juice
1/3 cup all-purpose flour
One Egg
Black pepper to taste
2 tsp olive oil

Directions :

Mesh beans in a large bowl using a potato masher, leave few whole beans according to need. Then add the garlic powder, onion, thyme, chipotle pepper, rice, corn, bell pepper, egg, flour, and lemon & mix well. Flavor with pepper. Make four patties of this mixture using hands. Take a large frying pan, add olive oil to it, and heat it on medium heat. For five minutes, cook burgers until browned onoone side, then flip its side and cook the other side for an additional 5 minutes.

Nutrition Info: Calories: 290 kcal Fat: 4 g Protein: 11 g Carbs: 50 g Fiber: 5 g

Chicken N' Orange Salad Sandwich

Preparation time: 5 minutes
Cooking time: 0 minute
Servings: 6

Ingredients:
1 cup Sliced cooked chicken
½ cup Chopped celery
½ cup Chopped green pepper
¼ cup chopped onion
1 cup Mandarin oranges
1/3 cup Mayonnaise

Directions :
Toss green pepper, chicken, onion & celery to combine. Add mayonnaise & mandarin oranges. Combine lightly. Enjoy with bread

Nutrition Info: Calories: 403 kcal Fat: 20 g Protein: 31 g Carbs: 24 g Fiber: 5 g

Avocado toast

Preparation time: 5 minutes
Cooking time: 2 minutes
Servings: 1

Ingredients:
Two slices of bread
½ sliced avocado
One pinch of Red pepper flakes
Sea salt
lemon or lime

Directions :
Toast the bread . Top the toasted bread with avocado (mashed or sliced). Sprinkle sea salts or red pepper flakes (according to taste)

Nutrition Info: Calories: 237 kcal Fat: 15.8 g Protein: 6.1 g Carbs: 21.2 g Fiber: 8.6 g

Overnight Oats

Preparation time: 7 minutes
Cooking time: 0 minute
Servings: 2

Ingredients:
1.5 cups Rolled Oats
1 cup Tinned coconut milk
1.5 cup Almond Milk
2 tbsp Chia Seeds
½ tsp Ground Cinnamon

Directions : Blend all the ingredients.

Nutrition Info: Calories: 256 kcal Fat: 6.9 g Protein: 11.4 g Carbs: 37.2 g Fiber: 6.6 g

Mjadera

Preparation time: 7 minutes

Cooking time: 0 minute

Servings: 4

Ingredients:

1 Cup Brown lentils

1 cup Bulgur

One Chopped Onion

2 tbsp Avocado or grapeseed oil

1/4 cup olive oil

Salt

Directions : Wash lentils & crook in the pot along with three cups water on moderate heat for fifteen minutes. Lentils should be dente. When lentils are cooking, cut the onion into dices and sauté with cooking oil and sauté and oil in a pan till brown. The darker the onion, is more flavorful the dish will be. Add uncooked bulgur, caramelized onion, one-fourth cup of olive oil, 1 cup water & salt according to taste. These are added into semi-cooked lentils on moderate heat till they are cooked fully. If the water dries and still lentils aren't cooked properly, add water according to need and cook again.

Nutrition Info: Calories: 534.4 kcal Fat: 22.1 g Protein: 17.3 g Carbs: 69.1 g Fiber: 10.6 g

Cabbage slaw

Preparation time: 7 minutes
Cooking time: 0 minute
Servings: 3

Ingredients:
3 cups Chopped Green Cabbage
2 cups Chopped Red Cabbage
2 cups Chopped Carrots
½ cup Chopped Cilantro
4 tbsp Lime Juice
3 tbsp Olive Oil

Directions :
Combine the ingredients all together in the bowl & toss them until the good mix
Prepare almost one-two hours ahead for the cabbage to soften & flavor to come together.

Nutrition Info: Calories: 118 kcal Fat: 3.5 g Protein: 17 g Carbs: 279 g Fiber: 27 g

Roasted grape crostini with ricotta and balsamic reduction

Preparation time: 10 minutes
Cooking time: 10 minutes
Servings: 4

Ingredients:

1/3 cup Balsamic vinegar
3 tbsp Olive oil
1 tsp Brown sugar
1 tsp fresh thyme
½ tsp Black pepper
½ lb Juicy seedless grapes
6 oz Ricotta or Mascarpone cheese
12 sliced of bread

Directions :

Preheat microwave to 400.
On a baking sheet, toss grape with thyme & 2 tbsp of olive oil. Season with pepper and toss to coat. Roast for almost 15 min. Occasionally stir till the grapes are fully softened. Brush baguette slices with 1tbsp of olive oil. Arrange them on a baking sheet & toast for 8 min till they become golden & crisp. When grapes are being roasted, reduce the vinegar on moderate heat till it thickens & reduce to two tbsp. Stir it in brown sugar & sprinkle it with black pepper. For assembling the crostini, dollop

half tbsp of ricotta cheese on a toast. Spoon the warm grapes on top & drizzle it with reduction. Garnish the dish with chopped rosemary.

Nutrition Info: Calories: 96 kcal Fat: 3 g Protein: 6 g Carbs: 13 g Fiber: 2 g

Low sodium herbed grilled corn

Preparation time: 3 minutes

Cooking time: 20 minutes

Servings: 3

Ingredients:

½ cup Unsalted butter

2 tbsp chopped parsley

2 tbsp chopped chives

1 tsp dried thyme

½ tsp Cayenne pepper

Eight Sweet corn

two limes

Directions :

Take a small bowl. Beat 1st five ingredients till they are fully blended. Spread one tbsp mixture on each ear of corn. Wrap the corn individually into the heavy foil. Grill the corn and cover it properly. Heat it for 15 min on moderate heat till it is tendered. Open the foil carefully to allow the steam to escape.

Nutrition Info: Calories: 182.3 kcal Fat: 12.6 g Protein: 3 g Carbs: 18 g Fiber: 2.5 g

Sour candy Grapes

Preparation time: 1 minute
Cooking time: 7 minutes
Servings: 3

Ingredients:
One box Gelatin per
3 lb of grapes
1 cup Water
Lemon juice

Directions :
Pour the gelatin into the small bowl.
Poke the toothpick in through a spot where the stem was connected.
With the help of a toothpick, dip it in the water & roll.
Put this into the refrigerator until chilled properly.
Once they are chilled, toothpicks can easily be removed.
Serve and enjoy the food.

Nutrition Info: Calories: 67 kcal Fat: 0 g Protein: 0.8 g Carbs: 18 g Fiber: 0.1 g

Incredible raspberry pear sorbet

Preparation time: 5 minutes
Cooking time: 20 minutes
Servings: 6 persons

Ingredients:
Half cup of sugar.
One pint of fresh raspberries.
1/3 cup lemon juice.
Two large pears.
1 tbsp of pear liqueur

Directions :
Simply take 1 cup of water into a pan. Add sugar to boil and wait till the sugar is dissolved completely. Reduce heat. Simmer it, uncovered for 3 min. Remove it from heat & place it in the refrigerator to cool. Meanwhile, combine one pint of raspberries, lime juice, pear & pear liqueur in a food processor. Now cover it and process until the mixture becomes soft and smooth. Prepare as ice cream maker instructions. Cover it, let it be freed for 4 hours or till it is completely solid. Then break the mixture with a fork & serve it with some extra raspberries.

Nutrition Info: Calories: 135 kcal Fat: 0.4 g Protein: 0.9 g Carbs: 31.7 g Fiber: 5 g

Cherry brown butter bars

Preparation time: 5 minutes
Cooking time: 40 minutes
Servings: 3

Ingredients:
Crust
¾ cup melted butter
2/3 cup sugar
½ tsp Vanilla extract
2.25 cups Flour
1/8 tsp Salt
Creamy Top and Cherry Filling
1 cup Grated unsalted butter
Three Eggs
2/3 cup Sugar
1/8 tsp Salt
½ cup Flour
1 tsp Vanilla extract
1 tsp Almond extract
4 cups Cherries

Directions :
Preheat the oven up to 374 & take a baking dish along with parchment paper.

Mix sugar, vanilla, butter in a pan on moderate heat. Continue to stir until it gives foam type look, turn clear & then becomes deep brown. Now put the butter into a glass. Now whisk together the eggs, sugar & salt in a medium bowl till the mixture is fully blended. Put the cherries in an arrangement on a cooled crust & pour the filling over the fruit carefully. Now bake for thirty minutes till the filling is golden and becomes puffed. If a toothpick is inserted in it, it should be so that it comes out dried and clean. Store these bars in the container for one day and then place them in the fridge.

Nutrition Info: Calories: 190 kcal Fat: 11 g Protein: 1 g Carbs: 22 g Fiber: 1 g

Honey garlic kebab marinade

Preparation time: 8 minutes
Cooking time: 15 minutes
Servings: 25 kebab

Ingredients:
¼ cup Olive oil
1/3 cup Honey
¼ cup Bragg's Liquid Aminos
¼ tsp Black pepper
3 Chopped garlic cloves

Directions :
Combine all ingredients in a plastic bag and mix properly. Add meat in it to marinate for 30 minutes overnight. Use marinade to baste kebabs for the first five min of cooking.

Nutrition Info: Calories: 645 kcal Fat: 19 g Protein: 52 g Carbs: 68 g Fiber: 5 g

Grilled blackened tilapia

Preparation time: 5 minutes
Cooking time: 10 minutes
Servings: 3

Ingredients:
Four filets of tilapia
2 tsp of smoked paprika
One tsp of dried oregano
1 tsp of garlic powder
3/4 tsp cumin
Half tsp of cayenne pepper
Two tbsp of olive oil

Directions :
Prepare the grill for moderate heat & lightly oil the grill grate. Pat fish to dry Mix the seasoning & coat the fish. Grill the fish for almost three min or till it is flaked easily. Garnish the dish with cilantro & serve.

Nutrition Info: Calories: 154 kcal Fat: 5 g Protein: 23 g Carbs: 4 g Fiber: 1 g

Zucchini and Feta Cake

Preparation time: 15 minutes
Cooking time: 45 minutes
Servings: 6

Ingredients:
Three zucchinis cubed
3 tbsp olive oil
One shallot shopped
Four eggs, whipped
250 gr flour
One pack of baking powder
50 ml of milk
2 cups basil leaves, thin strips
200 gr feta cubed
12 olives black, cut in half
salt & pepper

Directions :
Heat some olive oil in a frypan.
Pans fry the zucchini with shallot for around 10 minutes. Now season with salt & pepper. Preheat oven to the temperature of 180 ° C.
Add flour, baking powder, and whipped eggs in a bowl and combine. Then transfer olive oil &milk, again mix until a smooth

texture is obtained. Add zucchini, olives, basil & feta. Combine. Oil a cake tin, then pour preparation in & bake for around 40 minutes.
Serve

Nutrition Info: Calories: 1844 kcal Fat: 8g Protein: 915.57mg Carbs:21 g

Steamed Vegetables served with Macadamia Dressing

Preparation time: 15 minutes

Cooking time: 60 minutes

Servings: 2

Ingredients:

1/2 fennel bulb, cut into slices

1/2 pound trimmed asparagus

1/4 pound trimmed green beans

1/2 pound scrubbed small carrots

Dressing

3 tbsp fresh citrus juice

1 tsp raw apple cider vinegar

1/2 tsp honey

2 tbsp olive oil

1 1/2 tbsp fresh dill, chopped

1 1/2 tbsp f parsley, chopped

Four basil leaves, sliced

1/4 cup macadamia nuts, finely chopped

Salt coarse

Directions :

Mix the dressing ingredients in a bowl & season with some salt. Work in batches now steams vegetables till crisp and tender, 2 - 4 minutes.

Display vegetables on the platter, then season with salt and garnish with
dressing.

Nutrition Info: Calories:228 kcal Fat:1 g Protein: 13 g Carbs: 29 g Fiber:9 g

Broccoli a la Polonaise

Preparation time: 15 minutes
Cooking time: 15 minutes
Servings: 4

Ingredients:
One broccoli, florets cut
2 tbsp butter
½ cup breadcrumbs
1 tbsp Parmesan cheese, grated
One boiled egg, chopped

Directions :
Place the steamer, insert it in a saucepan, & fill with water below the steamer's bottom. Cover boil on high heat. Transfer the broccoli, cover, & steam till tender, 2 - 6 minutes, depends on thickness.
Melt the butter in a saucepan; add bread crumbs & Parmesan cheese, & cook until crumbs become golden brown, 1 - 2 minutes. Now sprinkle browned crumbs onto steamed broccoli, & toss gently. Sprinkle broccoli with the chopped egg.

Nutrition Info: Calories:166 kcal Fat:8.5 g Protein: 5.1g Carbs:17.4 g Fiber:3.6 g

Broccoli, cauliflower & feta salad

Preparation time: 25 minutes
Cooking time: 5 minutes
Servings: 6

Ingredients:
4 cups fresh broccoli
4 cups fresh cauliflower
1 cup raisins
One sliced red onion
1⁄2 cup almonds sliced
1 cup feta cheese crumbled
salt & black pepper
1 cup yogurt
4 tbsp sugar
1⁄2 cup mayonnaise
2 tbsp lemon juice

Directions : Mix mayonnaise sugar, yogurt & lemon juice; mix until completely combined. A separate glass bowl mix together broccoli & cauliflower florets, almonds, onion, raisins & feta cheese. Then pour dressing, then toss till combine. Sprinkle salt & pepper. Chill for 2 hours. Serve.

Nutrition Info: Calories: 344.3 kcal Fat:17.4 g Protein: 10.4 g Carbs:42.2 g Fiber: 3.6 g

Lentils, Zucchini & Tomato Sauce

Preparation time: 15 minutes
Cooking time: 30 minutes
Servings: 4

Ingredients:

2 ½ cup water

1 cup green lentils

1 tbsp olive oil

One cubed zucchini

½ diced large onion

Two minced cloves of garlic

2 tbsp chopped lavage

1 tbsp chopped thyme

2 cups tomato sauce

Directions : Bring lentils to a boil in a saucepan. Cover and simmer until tender for about 20 minutes. Heat olive oil in a skillet on high heat. Sauté onion, garlic, zucchini for 5 - 7 minutes. Add lavage & thyme & cook till slightly wilted 10 seconds. Add lentils & tomato sauce. Reduce heat & cook for 3 - 5 minutes.

Nutrition Info: Calories:288 kcal Fat:10.5 g Protein:11 g Carbs: 39 g Fiber:10 g

Pumpkin with Butternut Curry

Preparation time: 15 minutes

Cooking time: 25 minutes

Servings: 4

Ingredients:

5 cup pumpkin cubed

2 cups of water

1 tsp turmeric

salt

½ cup coconut grated

Three Chile peppers red

One Chile pepper green

2 tbsp water

1 tsp cumin seeds

1 tbsp coconut oil

Two red Chile peppers dried

1 tsp mustard seeds

1 tsp black lentils

1 tbsp coconut grated

Six curry leaves

Directions :

Add pumpkin, water, turmeric & salt in a pan and bring to boil & cook till pumpkin is tender about 15 minutes. Mix coconut, green Chile pepper, red Chile peppers, 2 tbsp water, & cumin seeds in the food processor and stir into pumpkin mixture. Cook till thickened & coats pumpkin cubes, 5 - 7 minutes. Pour in the serving bowl. Heat coconut oil in a small skillet, cook red Chile peppers, black lentils & mustard seeds until they sputter, for 2 - 3 minutes; pour it over a curry. Heat the remaining tsp coconut oil in a skillet. Heat coconut in hot oil until browned, 3 - 5 minutes. Pour on the curry. Serve

Nutrition Info: Calories:175 kcal Fat:12.6 g Protein: 3.5g Carbs:16 g Fiber: 3.5g

Simple Sautéed Cauliflower

Preparation time: 15 minutes

Cooking time: 15 minutes

Servings: 4

Ingredients:

One onion chopped

One head of cauliflower

¼ cup olive oil

1 cup cherry tomatoes

2 tbsp 1raisins

1 tsp white sugar

One minced garlic clove

1 tsp dried parsley

¼ tsp red pepper flakes

1 tbsp lemon juice

Directions :

Heat some olive oil in a wide skillet on medium heat; cook and mix in the onion until soft. 5-10 minutes are enough. Add the cauliflower, the cherry tomatoes, raisins, and finally white sugar to the onion; cover the skillet and roast, and stir regularly until the cauliflower is soft, for 4-5 minutes. Mix the garlic, parsley, and some red pepper flakes in the cauliflower mixture; heat up to maximum and Sautee them until the cauliflower gets browned for 1 to 3 minutes. Drizzle the juice of the lemon over the cauliflower.

Nutrition Info: Calories: 196.5kcal Fat: 13.9g Protein: 3.7g Carbs: 17.8g Fiber: 4.8g

BREAKFAST & LUNCH

Egg, Prosciutto, And Cheese Freezer Sandwiches

Servings: 6
Cooking Time: 20 Minutes

Ingredients:

Cooking spray or oil to grease the baking dish

7 large eggs

½ cup low-fat (2%) milk

½ teaspoon garlic powder

½ teaspoon onion powder

1 tablespoon Dijon mustard

½ teaspoon honey

6 whole-wheat English muffins

6 slices thinly sliced prosciutto

6 slices Swiss cheese

Directions:

Preheat the oven to 375°F. Lightly oil or spray an 8-by--inch glass or ceramic baking dish with cooking spray.

In a large bowl, whisk together the eggs, milk, garlic powder, and onion powder. Pour the mixture into the baking dish and bake for minutes, until the eggs are set and no longer jiggling. Cool.

While the eggs are baking, mix the mustard and honey in a small bowl. Lay out the English muffin halves to start assembly.

When the eggs are cool, use a biscuit cutter or drinking glass about the same size as the English muffin diameter to cut 6 egg circles. Divide the leftover egg scraps evenly to be added to each sandwich.

Spread ½ teaspoon of honey mustard on each of the bottom English muffin halves. Top each with 1 slice of prosciutto, 1 egg circle and scraps, 1 slice of cheese, and the top half of the muffin. Wrap each sandwich tightly in foil.

STORAGE: Store tightly wrapped sandwiches in the freezer for up to 1 month. To reheat, remove the foil, place the sandwich on a microwave-safe plate, and wrap with a damp paper towel. Microwave on high for 1½ minutes, flip over, and heat again for another 1½ minutes. Because cooking time can vary greatly between microwaves, you may need to experiment with a few sandwiches before you find the perfect amount of time to heat the whole item through.

Nutrition Info: Total calories: 361; Total fat: 17g; Saturated fat: 7g; Sodium: 953mg; Carbohydrates: 26g; Fiber: 3g; Protein:

Veggie Mediterranean Quiche

Servings: 8

Cooking Time: 55 Minutes

Ingredients:

1/2 cup sundried tomatoes - dry or in olive oil*

Boiling water

1 prepared pie crust

2 tbsp vegan butter

1 onion, diced

2 cloves garlic, minced

1 red pepper, diced

1/4 cup sliced Kalamata olives

1 tsp dried oregano

1 tsp dried parsley

1/3 cup crumbled feta cheese

4 large eggs

1 1/4 cup milk

2 cups fresh spinach or 1/2 cup frozen spinach, thawed and squeezed dry

Salt, to taste

Pepper, to taste

1 cup shredded cheddar cheese, divided

Directions:

If you're using dry sundried tomatoes - In a measure cup, add the sundried tomatoes and pour the boiling water over until just covered, allow to sit for 5 minutes or until the tomatoes are soft. The drain and chop tomatoes, set aside

Preheat oven to 375 degrees F

Fit a 9-inch pie plate with the prepared pie crust, then flute edges, and set aside

In a skillet over medium high heat, melt the butter

Add in the onion and garlic, and cook until fragrant and tender, about 3 minutes

Add in the red pepper, cook for an additional 3 minutes, or until the peppers are just tender

Add in the spinach, olives, oregano, and parsley, cook until the spinach is wilted (if you're using fresh) or heated through (if you're using frozen), about 5 minutes

Remove the pan from heat, stir in the feta cheese and tomatoes, spoon the mixture into the prepared pie crust, spreading out evenly, set aside

In a medium-sized mixing bowl, whisk together the eggs, 1/2 cup of the cheddar cheese, milk, salt, and pepper

Pour this egg and cheese mixture evenly over the spinach mixture in the pie crust

Sprinkle top with the remaining cheddar cheese

Bake for 50-55 minutes, or until the crust is golden brown and the egg is set

Allow to cool completely before slicing

Wrap the slices in plastic wrap and then aluminum foil and place in the freezer.

To Serve: Remove the aluminum foil and plastic wrap, and microwave for 2 minutes, then allow to rest for 30 seconds, enjoy!

Recipe Notes: You'll find two types of sundried tomatoes available in your local grocery store—dry ones and ones packed in olive oil. Both will work for this recipe.

If you decide to use dry ones, follow the directions in the recipe to reconstitute them. If you're using oil-packed sundried tomatoes, skip the first step and just remove them from the oil, chop them, and continue with the recipe.

Season carefully! Between the feta, cheddar, and olives, this recipe is naturally salty.

Nutrition Info: Calories:239; Carbs: Total Fat: 15g; Protein: 7g

Mediterranean Scrambled Eggs

Servings: 2
Cooking Time: 10 Minutes

Ingredients:

1 tbsp oil
1 yellow pepper, diced
2 spring onions, sliced
8 cherry tomatoes, quartered
2 tbsp sliced black olives
1 tbsp capers
4 eggs
1/4 tsp dried oregano
Black pepper
Topping:
Fresh parsley, to serve

Directions:

In a frying pan over medium heat, add the oil
Once heated, add the diced pepper and chopped spring onions, cook for a few minutes, until slightly soft
Add in the quartered tomatoes, olives and capers, and cook for 1 more minute
Crack the eggs into the pan, immediately scramble with a spoon or spatula

Sprinkle with oregano and plenty of black pepper, and stir until the eggs are fully cooked

Distribute the eggs evenly into the containers, store in the fridge for 2-3 days

To Serve: Reheat in the microwave for 30 seconds or in a toaster oven until warmed through

Nutrition Info: Calories:249;Carbs: 13g;Total Fat: 17g;Protein: 14g

Chia Pudding

Servings: 2

Cooking Time: 15 Minutes

Ingredients:

½ cup chia seeds

2 cups milk

1 tablespoon honey

Directions:

Combine and mix the chia seeds, milk, and honey in a bowl.

Put the mixture in the freezer and let it set.

Take the pudding out of the freezer only when you see that the pudding has thickened.

Serve chilled.

Nutrition Info: Calories: 429, Total Fat: 22.4g, Saturated Fat: 4.9, Cholesterol: 20 mg, Sodium: 124 mg, Total Carbohydrate: 44.g, Dietary Fiber: 19.5 g, Total Sugars: 19.6 g, Protein: 17.4 g, Vitamin D: 1 mcg, Calcium: 648 mg, Iron: 4 mg, Potassium: 376 mg

Breakfast Rice Bowls

Servings: 4
Cooking Time: 8 Minutes

Ingredients:
1 cup of brown rice
1 tsp ground cinnamon
1/4 cup almonds, sliced
2 tbsp sunflower seeds
1/4 cup pecans, chopped
1/4 cup walnuts, chopped
2 cup unsweetened almond milk
Pinch of salt

Directions:
Spray instant pot from inside with cooking spray.
Add all ingredients into the instant pot and stir well.
Seal pot with lid and cook on high for 8 minutes.
Once done, allow to release pressure naturally for 5 minutes then release remaining using quick release. Remove lid.
Stir well and serve.

Nutrition Info: Calories: 291; Fat: 12 g; Carbohydrates: 40.1 g; Sugar: 0.4 g; Protein: 7.g; Cholesterol: 0 mg

Tahini Egg Salad With Pita

Servings: 4
Cooking Time: 12 Minutes

Ingredients:
4 large eggs
¼ cup freshly chopped dill
1 tablespoon plus 1 teaspoon unsalted tahini
2 teaspoons freshly squeezed lemon juice
⅛ teaspoon kosher salt
4 whole-wheat pitas, quartered

Directions:
Place the eggs in a saucepan and cover with water. Bring the water to a boil. As soon as the water starts to boil, place a lid on the pan and turn the heat off. Set a timer for minutes.
When the timer goes off, drain the hot water and run cold water over the eggs to cool.
When the eggs are cool, peel them, place the yolks in a medium bowl, and mash them with a fork. Then chop the egg whites.
Add the chopped egg whites, dill, tahini, lemon juice (to taste), and salt to the bowl, and mix to combine.
Place a heaping ⅓ cup of egg salad in each of 4 containers. Place the pita in 4 separate containers or resealable bags so that the bread does not get soggy.

STORAGE: Store covered containers in the refrigerator for up to 5 days.

Nutrition Info: Total calories: 242; Total fat: 10g; Saturated fat: 2g; Sodium: 300mg; Carbohydrates: 29g; Fiber: 5g; Protein: 13g.

Strawberry-mango Green Smoothie

Servings: 2
Cooking Time: 10 Minutes

Ingredients:

1½ cups low-fat (2%) milk

2 cups packed baby spinach leaves

½ cup sliced Persian or English cucumber, skin on

⅔ cup frozen strawberries

⅔ cup frozen mango chunks

1 medium very ripe banana, sliced (about ⅔ cup)

½ small avocado

1 teaspoon honey

Directions:

Place the milk, spinach, cucumber, strawberries, mango, banana, and avocado in a blender.

Blend until smooth and taste. If the smoothie isn't sweet enough, add the honey.

Distribute the smoothie between 2 to-go cups.

STORAGE: Store smoothie cups in the refrigerator for up to 3 days.

Nutrition Info: Total calories: 261; Total fat: 8g; Saturated fat: 2g; Sodium: 146mg; Carbohydrates: 40g; Fiber: ; Protein: 11g

Breakfast Taco Scramble

Servings: 4

Cooking Time: 1 Hour 25 Minutes

Ingredients:

8 large eggs, beaten

1/4 tsp seasoning salt

1 lb 99% lean ground turkey

2 tbsp Greek seasoning

1/2 small onion, minced

2 tbsp bell pepper, minced

4 oz. can tomato sauce

1/4 cup water

1/4 cup chopped scallions or cilantro, for topping

For the potatoes:

12 (1 lb) baby gold or red potatoes, quartered

4 tsp olive oil

3/4 tsp salt

1/2 tsp garlic powder

fresh black pepper, to taste

Directions:

In a large bowl, beat the eggs, season with seasoning salt

Preheat the oven to 4 degrees F

Spray a 9x12 or large oval casserole dish with cooking oil

Add the potatoes 1 tbsp oil, 3/teaspoon salt, garlic powder and black pepper and toss to coat

Bake for 4minutes to 1 hour, tossing every 15 minutes

In the meantime, brown the turkey in a large skillet over medium heat, breaking it up while it cooks

Once no longer pink, add in the Greek seasoning

Add in the bell pepper, onion, tomato sauce and water, stir and cover, simmer on low for about 20 minutes

Spray a different skillet with nonstick spray over medium heat

Once heated, add in the eggs seasoned with 1/4 tsp of salt and scramble for 2–3 minutes, or cook until it sets

Distribute 3/4 cup turkey and 2/3 cup eggs and divide the potatoes in each storage container, store for 3-4 days

To Serve: Reheat in the microwave for 1-minute (until 90% heated through) top with shredded cheese if desired, and chopped scallions

Nutrition Info: (¼ of a the scramble): Calories:450;Total Fat: 19g;Total Carbs: 24.5g;Fiber: 4g;Protein: 46g

Whole-wheat Pancakes With Spiced Peach And Orange Compote

Servings: 6

Cooking Time: 15 Minutes

Ingredients:

1½ cups whole-wheat flour

1 teaspoon baking powder

½ teaspoon baking soda

½ teaspoon ground cinnamon

⅛ teaspoon kosher salt

1 large egg

1 cup low-fat (2%) plain Greek yogurt

1 tablespoon honey

1 cup low-fat (2%) milk

2 teaspoons olive oil, divided

1 (10-ounce) package frozen sliced peaches

½ cup orange juice

¼ teaspoon pumpkin pie spice

Directions:

TO MAKE THE PANCAKES

Combine the flour, baking powder, baking soda, cinnamon, and salt in a large mixing bowl and whisk to make sure everything is distributed evenly. In a separate bowl, whisk together the egg, yogurt, honey, and milk. Pour the liquid ingredients into the dry ingredients and stir until just combined. Do not overmix.

Heat ½ teaspoon of oil in a 12-inch skillet or griddle over medium heat. Once the pan is hot, spoon ¼ cup of pancake batter into the pan. You should be able to fit pancakes in a 12-inch skillet. Cook each side for about 1 minute and 30 seconds, watching carefully and checking the underside for a golden but not burnt color before flipping. Repeat until all the batter has been used.

Place 2 pancakes in each of 6 containers.

TO MAKE THE COMPOTE

Thaw the peaches in the microwave just to the point that they can be cut, about 30 seconds on high. Cut the peaches into 1-inch pieces.

Bring the peaches, orange juice, and pumpkin pie spice to a boil in a saucepan. As soon as bubbles appear, lower the heat to medium-low and cook for 12 minutes, until the juice has thickened and the peaches are very soft. Allow to cool, then mash with a potato masher.

Place 2 tablespoons of compote in each of 6 sauce containers.

STORAGE: Store covered pancake containers in the refrigerator for up to 5 days or in the freezer for up to 2 months. Peach compote will last up to 2 weeks in the refrigerator and up to 2 months in the freezer.

Nutrition Info: Total calories: 209; Total fat: 5g; Saturated fat: 2g; Sodium: 289mg; Carbohydrates: 34g; Fiber: 4g; Protein: 11g

Peanut Butter Banana Greek Yogurt

Servings: 4

Cooking Time: 5 Minutes

Ingredients:

3 cups vanilla Greek yogurt

2 medium bananas sliced

1/4 cup creamy natural peanut butter

1/4 cup flaxseed meal

1 tsp nutmeg

Directions:

Divide yogurt between four jars with lids

Top with banana slices

In a bowl, melt the peanut butter in a microwave safe bowl for - 40 seconds and drizzle one tbsp on each bowl on top of the bananas

Store in the fridge for up to 3 days

When ready to serve, sprinkle with flaxseed meal and ground nutmeg

Enjoy!

Nutrition Info: Calories:3;Carbs: 47g;Total Fat: 10g;Protein: 22g

Green Shakshuka

Servings: 2

Cooking Time: 15 Minutes

Ingredients:

1 tbsp olive oil

1 onion, peeled and diced

1 clove garlic, peeled and finely minced

3 cups broccoli rabe, chopped

3 cups baby spinach leaves

2 tbsp whole milk or cream

1 tsp ground cumin

1/4 tsp black pepper

1/4 tsp salt (or to taste)

4 Eggs

Garnish:

1 pinch sea salt

1 pinch red pepper flakes

Directions:

Pre-heat the oven to 350 degrees F

Add the broccoli rabe to a large pot of boiling water, cook for minutes, drain and set aside

In a large oven-proof skillet or cast-iron pan over medium heat, add in the tablespoon of olive oil along with the diced onions, cook for about 10 minutes or until the onions become translucent

Add the minced garlic and continue cooking for about another minute

Cut the par-cooked broccoli rabe into small pieces, stir into the onion and garlic mixture

Cook for a couple of minutes, then stir in the baby spinach leaves, continue to cook for a couple more minutes, stirring often, until the spinach begins to wilt

Stir in the ground cumin, salt, ground black pepper, and milk

Make four wells in the mixture, crack an egg into each well – be careful not to break the yolks. Also, note that it's easier to crack each egg into a small bowl and then transfer them to the pan

Place the pan with the eggs into the pre-heated oven, cook for 10 to 15 minutes until the eggs are set to preference

Sprinkle the cooked eggs with a dash of sea salt and a pinch of red pepper flakes

Allow to cool, distribute among the containers, store for 2-3 days

To Serve: Microwave for 1-minute or until heated through, serve with crusty whole-wheat bread or warmed slices of pita or naan

Nutrition Info: Calories:278; Carbs: 18g;Total Fat: 16g;Protein: 16g

Clean Breakfast Cookies

Servings: 4
Cooking Time: 20 Minutes

Ingredients:
2 cups oats (rolled)
1 cup whole wheat flour
¼ cup flax seed
2½ teaspoons cinnamon (ground)
1 cup honey
½ teaspoon baking soda
2 egg whites
½ teaspoon vanilla extract
4 tablespoons almond butter
pinch of salt

Directions:
Preheat oven to 325 degrees F.
Whisk oats, flour, flaxseed, cinnamon, salt, and baking soda together in a bowl.
Then, stir honey, egg whites, almond butter, and vanilla extract into the oats mixture until dough is blended.
Now, prepare the baking sheets and scoop the dough in them.
Finally, bake for about 20 minutes.
Serve warm or room temperature.

Nutrition Info: Calories: 686, Total Fat: 14.3g, Saturated Fat: 1.3, Cholesterol: 0 mg, Sodium: 185 mg, Total Carbohydrate: 131.4 g, Dietary Fiber: 11.9 g, Total Sugars: .2 g, Protein: 15.6 g, Vitamin D: 0 mcg, Calcium: 100 mg, Iron: 9 mg, Potassium: 456 mg

Omelet With Cheese And Broccoli

Servings: 4

Cooking Time: 30 Minutes

Ingredients:

6 eggs

2 ½ cups of broccoli florets

¼ cup of milk

1 tablespoon olive oil

⅓ cup Romano cheese, grated

¼ teaspoon pepper

⅕ teaspoon salt

⅓ cup Greek olives, sliced

Parsley and more Romano cheese for garnish

Directions:

Turn your oven to broil.

Set a steamer basket in a large pan and add 1 inch of water.

Add the broccoli to the steamer basket and turn the range to medium. Once the water starts to boil, reduce the temperature to low. Steam the broccoli for 4 to 5 minutes. You will know the vegetable is done when it is soft and tender.

In a large bowl, whisk the eggs.

Pour in the milk, pepper, and salt.

Once the broccoli is done, toss into the large bowl and add the olives and grated cheese.

Grease an oven-proof 10-inch skillet and turn the heat on the burner to medium.

Add in the egg mixture, then cook for 4 to 5 minutes.

Set the skillet into the oven but make sure it's at least 4 inches from the heating source. Broil the eggs for 3 minutes. If the eggs are not completely set, continue cooking for another minute or two.

Remove the eggs from the oven and set on the stove so they can cool for a few minutes.

Garnish the omelet with cheese and parsley. Then, cut into wedges and enjoy!

Nutrition Info: calories: 229, fats: 17 grams, carbohydrates: 5 grams, protein: 15 grams.

Greek Yogurt Breakfast Bowl

Servings: 1

Cooking Time: 5 Minutes

Ingredients:

1 cup Greek Yogurt plain

13 cup Pomegranate Seeds (or fresh fruit of your choice)

1 tsp honey

Directions:

In a jar with a lid, add the Greek yogurt in a bowl top with fruit and drizzle honey over the top

Close the lid and refrigerate for 3 days

Nutrition Info: Calories116; Carbs 24g;Total Fat 1.2g;Protein 4g

Cucumber Celery Lime Smoothie

Servings: 2

Cooking Time: 15 Minutes

Ingredients:

8 stalks of celery, chopped

1 lemon, juiced

2 cucumbers, peeled and chopped

½ cup ice

sweetener of your choice

1 cup water

Directions:

Place all the Ingredients: in a blender.

Blend well until smooth and frothy or desired texture.

Serve chilled.

Enjoy.

Nutrition Info: Calories: 64, Total Fat: 0., Saturated Fat: 0.2, Cholesterol: 0 mg, Sodium: 63 mg, Total Carbohydrate: 15.7 g, Dietary Fiber: 3.4 g, Total Sugars: 6.7 g, Protein: 2.8 g, Vitamin D: 0 mcg, Calcium: 85 mg, Iron: 1 mg, Potassium: 660 mg

Chocolate-almond Banana Bread

Servings: 4

Cooking Time: 25 Minutes

Ingredients:

Cooking spray or oil to grease the pan

1 cup almond meal

2 large eggs

2 very ripe bananas, mashed

1 tablespoon plus 2 teaspoons maple syrup

½ teaspoon vanilla extract

½ teaspoon baking powder

¼ teaspoon ground cardamom

⅓ cup dark chocolate chips, very roughly chopped

Directions:

Preheat the oven to 350°F and spray an 8-inch cake pan or baking dish with cooking spray or rub with oil.

Combine all the ingredients in a large mixing bowl. Then pour the mixture into the prepared pan.

Place the pan in the oven and bake for 25 minutes. The edges should be browned, and a paring knife should come out clean when the banana bread is pierced.

When cool, slice into wedges and place 1 wedge in each of 4 containers.

STORAGE: Store covered containers at room temperature for up to 2 days, refrigerate for up to 7 days, or freeze for up to 3 months.

Nutrition Info: Total calories: 3; Total fat: 23g; Saturated fat: 6g; Sodium: 105mg; Carbohydrates: 37g; Fiber: 6g; Protein: 10g

Mediterranean Breakfast Egg White Sandwich

Servings: 1

Cooking Time: 30 Minutes

Ingredients:

1 tsp vegan butter

¼ cup egg whites

1 tsp chopped fresh herbs such as parsley, basil, rosemary

1 whole grain seeded ciabatta roll

1 tbsp pesto

1-2 slices muenster cheese (or other cheese such as provolone, Monterey Jack, etc.)

About ½ cup roasted tomatoes

Salt, to taste

Pepper, to taste

Roasted Tomatoes:

10 oz grape tomatoes

1 tbsp extra virgin olive oil

Kosher salt, to taste

Coarse black pepper, to taste

Directions:

In a small nonstick skillet over medium heat, melt the vegan butter

Pour in egg whites, season with salt and pepper, sprinkle with fresh herbs, cook for 3-4 minutes or until egg is done, flip once

In the meantime, toast the ciabatta bread in toaster

Once done, spread both halves with pesto

Place the egg on the bottom half of sandwich roll, folding if necessary, top with cheese, add the roasted tomatoes and top half of roll sandwich

To make the roasted tomatoes: Preheat oven to 400 degrees F. Slice tomatoes in half lengthwise. Then place them onto a baking sheet and drizzle with the olive oil, toss to coat. Season with salt and pepper and roast in oven for about 20 minutes, until the skin appears wrinkled.

Nutrition Info: Calories:458; Total Carbohydrates: 51g; Total Fat: 0g; Protein: 21g

Strawberry-apricot Smoothie

Servings: 2
Cooking Time: 15 Minutes

Ingredients:
1 cup strawberries, frozen
¾ cup almond milk, unsweetened
2 apricots, pitted and sliced

Directions:
Put all the Ingredients: into the blender.
Blend them for a minute or until you reach desired foamy texture.
Serve the smoothie.
Enjoy.

Nutrition Info: Calories: 247, Total Fat: 21.9 g, Saturated Fat: 19 g, Cholesterol: 0 mg, Sodium: 1mg, Total Carbohydrate: 14.4 g, Dietary Fiber: 4.1 g, Total Sugars: 9.7 g, Protein: 3 g, Vitamin D: 0 mcg, Calcium: 30 mg, Iron: 2 mg, Potassium: 438 mg

Apple Quinoa Breakfast Bars

Servings: 12

Cooking Time: 40 Minutes

Ingredients:

2 eggs

1 apple peeled and chopped into ½ inch chunks

1 cup unsweetened apple sauce

1 ½ cups cooked & cooled quinoa

1 ½ cups rolled oats

1/4 cup peanut butter

1 tsp vanilla

1/2 tsp cinnamon

1/4 cup coconut oil

½ tsp baking powder

Directions:

Heat oven to 350 degrees F

Spray an 8x8 inch baking dish with oil, set aside

In a large bowl, stir together the apple sauce, cinnamon, coconut oil, peanut butter, vanilla and eggs

Add in the cooked quinoa, rolled oats and baking powder, mix until completely incorporated

Fold in the apple chunks

Spread the mixture into the prepared baking dish, spreading it to each corner

Bake for 40 minutes, or until a toothpick comes out clean

Allow to cool before slicing

Wrap the bars individually in plastic wrap. Store in an airtight container or baggie in the freezer for up to a month.

To serve: Warm up in the oven at 350 F for 5 minutes or microwave for up to 30 seconds.

Nutrition Info: (1 bar): Calories:230;Total Fat: 10g;Total Carbs: 31g;Protein: 7g

Pepper, Kale, And Chickpea Shakshuka

Servings: 5

Cooking Time: 35 Minutes

Ingredients:

1 tablespoon olive oil

1 small red onion, thinly sliced

1 red bell pepper, thinly sliced

1 green bell pepper, thinly sliced

1 bunch kale, stemmed and roughly chopped

½ cup packed cilantro leaves, chopped

½ teaspoon kosher salt

1 teaspoon smoked paprika

1 (14.5-ounce) can diced tomatoes

1 (14-ounce) can low-sodium chickpeas, drained and rinsed

⅔ cup water

5 eggs

2½ whole-wheat pitas (optional)

Directions:

Preheat the oven to 375°F.

Heat the oil in an oven-safe 1inch skillet over medium-high heat. Once the oil is shimmering, add the onions and red and green bell peppers. Sauté for 5 minutes, then cover, leaving the lid slightly ajar. Cook for 5 more minutes, then add the kale and cover, leaving the lid slightly ajar. Cook for 10 more minutes, stirring occasionally.

Add the cilantro, salt, paprika, tomatoes, chickpeas, and water, and stir to combine.

Make 5 wells in the mixture. Break an egg into a small bowl and pour it into a well. Repeat with the remaining eggs.

Place the pan in the oven and bake until the egg whites are opaque and the eggs still jiggle a little when the pan is shaken, about 12 to 1minutes, but start checking at 8 minutes.

When the shakshuka is cool, scoop about 1¼ cups of veggies into each of 5 containers, along with 1 egg each. If using, place ½ pita in each of 5 resealable bags.

STORAGE: Store covered containers in the refrigerator for up to 5 days.

Nutrition Info: Total calories: 244; Total fat: 9g; Saturated fat: 2g; Sodium: 529mg; Carbohydrates: 29g; Fiber: ; Protein: 14g

Rosemary Broccoli Cauliflower Mash

Servings: 3

Cooking Time: 12 Minutes

Ingredients:

2 cups broccoli, chopped

1 lb cauliflower, cut into florets

1 tsp dried rosemary

1/4 cup olive oil

1 tsp garlic, minced

Salt

Directions: Add broccoli and cauliflower into the instant pot.
Pour enough water into the pot to cover broccoli and cauliflower.
Seal pot with lid and cook on high for 1minutes.
Once done, allow to release pressure naturally. Remove lid.
Drain broccoli and cauliflower well and clean the instant pot.
Add oil into the pot and set the pot on sauté mode.
Add broccoli, cauliflower, rosemary, garlic, and salt and cook for 10 minutes.
Mash the broccoli and cauliflower mixture using a potato masher until smooth. Serve and enjoy.

Nutrition Info: Calories: 205;Fat: 17.2 g; Carbohydrates: 12.6 g; Sugar: 4.7 g; Protein: 4.8 g; Cholesterol: 0 mg

Pumpkin, Apple, And Greek Yogurt Muffins

Servings: 12

Cooking Time: 20 Minutes

Ingredients:

Cooking spray to grease baking liners

2 cups whole-wheat flour

1 teaspoon aluminum-free baking powder (see tip)

1 teaspoon baking soda

⅛ teaspoon kosher salt

2 teaspoons ground cinnamon

½ teaspoon ground ginger

½ teaspoon ground allspice

⅔ cup pure maple syrup

1 cup low-fat (2%) plain Greek yogurt

1 cup 100% canned pumpkin

1 large egg

¼ cup extra-virgin olive oil

1½ cups chopped green apple (leave peel on)

½ cup walnut pieces

Directions:

Preheat the oven to 400°F and line a muffin tin with baking liners. Spray the liners lightly with cooking spray.

In a large bowl, whisk together the flour, baking powder, baking soda, salt, cinnamon, ginger, and allspice.

In a medium bowl, combine the maple syrup, yogurt, pumpkin, egg, olive oil, chopped apple, and walnuts.

Pour the wet ingredients into the dry ingredients and combine just until blended. Do not overmix.

Scoop about ¼ cup of batter into each muffin liner and bake for 20 minutes, or until the tops look browned and a paring knife comes out clean when inserted. Remove the muffins from the tin to cool.

STORAGE: Store covered containers at room temperature for up to 4 days. To freeze the muffins for up to 3 months, wrap them in foil and place in an airtight resealable bag.

Nutrition Info: Total calories: 221; Total fat: 9g; Saturated fat: 1g; Sodium: 18g; Carbohydrates: 32g; Fiber: 4g; Protein: 6g

Cocoa And Raspberry Overnight Oats

Servings: 5

Cooking Time: 10 Minutes

Ingredients:

1⅔ cups rolled oats

3⅓ cups unsweetened vanilla almond milk

2 teaspoons vanilla extract

1 tablespoon plus 2 teaspoons pure maple syrup

3 tablespoons chia seeds

3 tablespoons unsweetened cocoa powder

1⅔ cups frozen raspberries

5 teaspoons cocoa nibs (optional)

Directions:

In a large bowl, mix the oats, almond milk, vanilla, maple syrup, chia seeds, and cocoa powder until well combined.

Spoon ¾ cup of the oat mixture into each of 5 containers.

Top each serving with ⅓ cup of raspberries and 1 teaspoon of cocoa nibs, if using.

STORAGE: Store covered containers in the refrigerator for up to 5 days.

Nutrition Info: Total calories: 21 Total fat: 6g; Saturated fat: <1g; Sodium: 121mg; Carbohydrates: 34g; Fiber: 10g; Protein: 7g

Bacon Brie Omelet With Radish Salad

Servings: 6

Cooking Time: 10 Minutes

Ingredients:

200 g smoked lardons

3 teaspoons olive oil, divided

7 ounces smoked bacon

6 lightly beaten eggs

small bunch chives, snipped up

3½ ounces sliced brie

1 teaspoon red wine vinegar

1 teaspoon Dijon mustard

1 cucumber, deseeded, halved, and sliced up diagonally

7 ounces radish, quartered

Directions:

Heat up the grill.

Add 1 teaspoon of oil to a small pan and heat on the grill.

Add lardons and fry them until nice and crisp.

Drain the lardon on kitchen paper.

Heat the remaining 2 teaspoons of oil in a non-sticking pan on the grill.

Add lardons, eggs, chives, and ground pepper, and cook over low heat until semi-set.

Carefully lay the Brie on top, and grill until it has set and is golden in color.

Remove from pan and cut into wedges.

Make the salad by mixing olive oil, mustard, vinegar, and seasoning in a bowl.

Add cucumber and radish and mix well.

Serve the salad alongside the omelet wedges in containers.

Enjoy!

Nutrition Info: Calories: 620, Total Fat: 49.3g, Saturated Fat: 22.1, Cholesterol: 295 mg, Sodium: 1632 mg, Total Carbohydrate: 4.3g, Dietary Fiber: 0.9 g, Total Sugars: 2.5 g, Protein: 39.2 g, Vitamin D: 41 mcg, Calcium: 185 mg, Iron: 2 mg, Potassium: 527 mg

Cranberry Oatmeal

Servings: 2

Cooking Time: 6 Minutes

Ingredients:

1/2 cup steel-cut oats

1 cup unsweetened almond milk

1 1/2 tbsp maple syrup

1/4 tsp cinnamon

1/4 tsp vanilla

1/4 cup dried cranberries

1 cup of water

1 tsp lemon zest, grated

1/4 cup orange juice

Directions:

Add all ingredients into the heat-safe dish and stir well.

Pour 1 cup of water into the instant pot then place the trivet in the pot. Place dish on top of the trivet.

Seal pot with lid and cook on high for 6 minutes.

Once done, allow to release pressure naturally for 10 minutes then release remaining using quick release. Remove lid. Serve and enjoy.

Nutrition Info: Calories: 161;Fat: 3.2 g; Carbohydrates: 29.9 g; Sugar: 12.4 g; Protein: 3.4 g; Cholesterol: 0 mg

Ricotta Fig Toast

Servings: 1
Cooking Time: 15 Minutes

Ingredients:
2 slices whole-wheat toast
1 teaspoon honey
¼ cup ricotta (partly skimmed)
1 dash cinnamon
2 figs (sliced)
1 teaspoon sesame seeds

Directions:
Start by mixing ricotta with honey and dash of cinnamon.
Then, spread this mixture on the toast.
Now, top with fig and sesame seeds.
Serve.

Nutrition Info: Calories: 372, Total Fat: 8.8g, Saturated Fat: 3.8, Cholesterol: 19 mg, Sodium: 373 mg, Total Carbohydrate: .7 g, Dietary Fiber: 8.8 g, Total Sugars: 27.1 g, Protein: 17 g, Vitamin D: 0 mcg, Calcium: 328 mg, Iron: 3 mg, Potassium: 518 mg

Mushroom Goat Cheese Frittata

Servings: 4

Cooking Time: 35 Minutes

Ingredients:

1 tbsp olive oil

1 small onion, diced

10 oz crimini or your favorite mushrooms, sliced

1 garlic clove, minced

10 eggs

2/3 cup half and half

1/4 cup fresh chives, minced

2 tsp fresh thyme, minced

1/2 tsp kosher salt

1/2 tsp black pepper

4 oz goat cheese

Directions:

Preheat the oven to 375 degrees F

In an over safe skillet or cast-iron pan over medium heat, olive oil

Add in the onion and sauté for 5 mins until golden

Add in the sliced mushrooms and garlic, continue to sauté until mushrooms are golden brown, about 10-12 minutes

In a large bowl, whisk together the eggs, half and half, chives, thyme, salt and pepper

Place the goat cheese over the mushroom mixture and pour the egg mixture over the top

Stir the mixture in the pan and cook over medium heat until the edges are set but the center is still loose, about 8-10 minutes

Put the pan in the oven and finish cooking for an additional 10 minutes or until set

Allow to cool completely before slicing

Wrap the slices in plastic wrap and then aluminum foil and place in the freezer.

To Serve: Remove the aluminum foil and plastic wrap, and microwave for 2 minutes, then allow to rest for 30 seconds, enjoy!

Nutrition Info: Calories:243;Total Carbohydrates: 5g;Total Fat: 17g;Protein: 15g

Honey, Dried Apricot, And Pistachio Yogurt Parfait

Servings: 3
Cooking Time: 10 Minutes

Ingredients:

1 (16-ounce) container low-fat (2%) plain Greek yogurt

1 tablespoon honey

½ teaspoon rose water (optional)

½ cup unsalted shelled pistachios, roughly chopped

12 dried apricot halves, quartered

Directions:

Mix the yogurt, honey, and rose water (if using) in a medium bowl.

Place ⅔ cup of yogurt in each of 3 containers. Top each mound of yogurt with equal portions of the pistachios and apricots.

STORAGE: Store covered containers in the refrigerator for up to 7 days.

Nutrition Info: Total calories: 275; Total fat: 12g; Saturated fat: 3g; Sodium: 72mg; Carbohydrates: 26g; Fiber: 3g; Protein: 19g

Mediterranean Stuffed Sweet Potatoes With Chickpeas And Avocado Tahini

Servings: 4

Cooking Time: 40 Minutes

Ingredients:

8 medium sized sweet potatoes, rinsed well

Marinated Chickpeas:

1 (15 oz) can chickpeas, drained and rinsed

1/2 red pepper, diced

3 tbsp extra virgin olive oil

1 tbsp fresh lemon juice

1 tbsp lemon zest

1 clove;about 1/2 teaspoon garlic, crushed

1 tbsp freshly chopped parsley

1 tbsp fresh oregano

1/4 tsp sea salt

Avocado Tahini Sauce:

1 medium sized ripe avocado

1/4 cup tahini

1/4 cup water

1 clove garlic, crushed

1 tbsp fresh parsley

1 tbsp fresh lemon juice

Toppings:

1/4 cup pepitas, hulled pumpkin seeds

Crumbled vegan feta or regular feta

Directions:

Preheat the oven to 400 degrees F

With a fork to pierce a few holes in the sweet potatoes

Place them on a baking sheet and bake for 45 minutes to an hour, or until the potatoes are tender to the touch. (Note that larger sweet potato will take longer to bake)

In the meantime, prepare the chickpeas by placing them in a medium sized bowl, combine the chickpeas with the extra virgin olive oil, lemon juice, lemon zest, red bell peppers, garlic, parsley, oregano, and sea salt. Toss the chickpeas until they're all coated in the marinade, set aside

Avocado Tahini Sauce:

Create the sauce by adding the ripe avocado, tahini, water, garlic, parsley, and lemon juice into a blender and process until smooth - If you would like a thinned consistency add another 1-2 tbsp of water

Once smooth transfer the sauce to a small bowl, set aside

To Assembly:

Once the sweet potatoes are tender, remove them from the oven and set aside until they are cool enough to handle

Then cut a slit down the middle of each potato and carefully spoon the chickpeas inside

Place the potato and chickpeas bake into container, store for 2-3 days

To Serve: Heat through in the oven at 374 degrees F for 5-8 minutes or until heated through. Top with the avocado tahini and sprinkle the pepitas and crumbled feta. Enjoy

Recipe Notes: There will be leftover chickpeas & avocado tahini - save the extras to make more sweet potatoes or create a big salad for a different lunch

Nutrition Info: Calories:308;Carbs: 38g;Total Fat: 15g;Protein: 7g

Walnut Banana Oatmeal

Servings: 2

Cooking Time: 3 Minutes

Ingredients:

1/2 cup steel-cut oats

1 cup of water

1 cup unsweetened almond milk

1 tsp honey

2 tbsp walnuts, chopped

1/2 banana, chopped

Directions:

Spray instant pot from inside with cooking spray.

Add oats, water, and almond milk into the instant pot and stir well.

Seal pot with lid and cook on high for minutes.

Once done, release pressure using quick release. Remove lid.

Stir in honey, walnut, and banana and serve.

Nutrition Info: Calories: 183; Fat: 7.8 g; Carbohydrates: 25.2 g; Sugar: 8 g; Protein: 5.4 g; Cholesterol: 0 mg

Super-seed Granola

Servings: 8
Cooking Time: 40 Minutes

Ingredients:
1½ cups rolled oats
⅓ cup raw quinoa
⅓ cup green pumpkin seeds (pepitas)
⅓ cup raw, unsalted sunflower seeds
2 tablespoons chia seeds
1 teaspoon ground cinnamon
⅓ cup pure maple syrup
⅓ cup unsweetened, unsalted sunflower seed butter

Directions:
Preheat the oven to 325°F. Line a baking sheet with a silicone mat or parchment paper.
In a large mixing bowl, combine the oats, quinoa, pumpkin seeds, sunflower seeds, chia seeds, and cinnamon.
Place the maple syrup and sunflower seed butter in a small microwaveable bowl and microwave for 20 seconds to melt the seed butter. Pour it over the oat mixture and stir to coat.
Spread the granola evenly across the lined pan, bake for 15 minutes, stir, bake for 15 more minutes, stir, and bake for 10 more minutes. Remove the granola from the oven; it will get crunchier as it cools.

Place ½ cup of granola in each of 8 containers and store at room temperature.

STORAGE: Store covered containers at room temperature for 2 weeks.

Nutrition Info: Total calories: 258; Total fat: 13g; Saturated fat: 1g; Sodium: 19mg; Carbohydrates: 30g; Fiber: 4g; Protein: 9g

Ham And Egg Muffins

Servings: 6

Cooking Time: 25 Minutes

Ingredients:

¼ cup crumbled feta cheese

⅛ teaspoon salt

1 ½ tablespoons of pesto sauce

9 slices of deli ham

⅓ cup chopped spinach

5 eggs

⅛ teaspoon of pepper

½ cup roasted red pepper plus a little for garnish

Basil for garnish

Directions:

Turn the temperature on your oven to 400 degrees Fahrenheit.

Grease the cups of the muffin tin.

Line each muffin tin cup with a slice of ham. The trick is to ensure there are no holes within the ham so none of the egg mixture seeps out.

Add some roasted peppers into the muffin cup.

Add 1 tablespoon of chopped spinach on top of the roasted pepper.

Sprinkle ½ tablespoon of feta cheese on top of the spinach.

Combine the eggs in a bowl with the salt and pepper. Whisk well.

Divide the egg mixture evenly between the 6 muffin tins.

Set in your oven and turn the timer for 15 minutes. If the eggs are not set and puffy after 15 minutes, keep them in the oven for another minute or two.

Carefully remove the muffins from the muffin tin cups and let them cool completely.

Garnish and enjoy your breakfast muffins, or you can store them in the fridge for up to three days. To warm them up, microwave them for 30 seconds.

Nutrition Info: calories: 109, fats: 6 grams, carbohydrates: 2 grams, protein: 9 grams.

Almond Pancakes

Servings: 6

Cooking Time: 30 Minutes

Ingredients:

½ cup melted coconut oil, plus a little on the side for grease

2 cups unsweetened, room temperature almond milk

2 teaspoons raw honey

1 ½ cups whole wheat flour

2 eggs, room temperature

¼ teaspoon ground cinnamon

½ cup almond flour

¼ teaspoon sea salt

½ teaspoon baking soda

1 ½ teaspoons baking powder

Directions:

In a large bowl, whisk your eggs.

Add in the coconut oil, honey, and almond milk. Whisk thoroughly.

In a separate bowl, sift together your baking soda, baking powder, sea salt, almond flour, cinnamon, and whole wheat flour. Ensure the ingredients are well incorporated.

Combine the two mixtures by slowly adding your powdered ingredients into your wet ingredients. Stir as you combine as it will be easier to fully mix the ingredients.

Grease a large skillet with oil and set it on medium-high heat.

Using ½ cup measurements, pour the batter into the skillet. Make sure the pancakes are not touching each other when they cook.

Let your pancakes cook for about 3 to 5 minutes on each side. Once bubbles start to break the surface and the edges become firm, flip the pancake over to cook the other side.

Once they are cooked thoroughly, place them on a plate and continue the process until all your batter is used up. You might need to grease your skillet again between batches.

To give your pancakes more of a Mediterranean flavor, add some fresh fruit on top.

Nutrition Info: calories: 286, fats: 17 grams, carbohydrates: 26 grams, protein: 7 grams.

Mediterranean Egg Muffins With Ham

Servings: 6
Cooking Time: 15 Minutes

Ingredients:
9 Slices of thin cut deli ham
1/2 cup canned roasted red pepper, sliced + additional for garnish
1/3 cup fresh spinach, minced
1/4 cup feta cheese, crumbled
5 large eggs
Pinch of salt
Pinch of pepper
1 1/2 tbsp Pesto sauce
Fresh basil for garnish

Directions:
Preheat oven to 400 degrees F
Spray a muffin tin with cooking spray, generously
Line each of the muffin tin with 1 ½ pieces of ham - making sure there aren't any holes for the egg mixture come out of
Place some of the roasted red pepper in the bottom of each muffin tin
Place 1 tbsp of minced spinach on top of each red pepper
Top the pepper and spinach off with a large 1/2 tbsp of crumbled feta cheese

In a medium bowl, whisk together the eggs salt and pepper, divide the egg mixture evenly among the 6 muffin tins

Bake for 15 to 17 minutes until the eggs are puffy and set

Remove each cup from the muffin tin

Allow to cool completely

Distribute the muffins among the containers, store in the fridge for 2 - 3days or in the freezer for 3 months

To Serve: Heat in the microwave for 30 seconds or until heated through. Garnish with 1/4 tsp pesto sauce, additional roasted red pepper slices and fresh basil.

Nutrition Info: Calories:109;Carbs: 2g;Total Fat: 6g;Protein: 9g

Overnight Berry Chia Oats

Servings: 1

Cooking Time: 5 Minutes

Ingredients:

1/2 cup Quaker Oats rolled oats

1/4 cup chia seeds

1 cup milk or water

pinch of salt and cinnamon

maple syrup, or a different sweetener, to taste

1 cup frozen berries of choice or smoothie leftovers

Toppings:

Yogurt

Berries

Directions:

In a jar with a lid, add the oats, seeds, milk, salt, and cinnamon, refrigerate overnight.

On serving day, puree the berries in a blender

Stir the oats, add in the berry puree and top with yogurt and more berries, nuts, honey, or garnish of your choice. Enjoy!

Recipe Notes: Make 3 jars at a time in individual jars for easy grab and go breakfasts for the next few days.

Nutrition Info: Calories:405;Carbs: g; Total Fat: 11g;Protein: 17g ù

Quinoa

Servings: 4

Cooking Time: 8 Hours

Ingredients:

1 cup quinoa (uncooked)

2 cups water

1 tablespoon raw honey

1 cup coconut milk

Topping(s) of your preference (nuts, cinnamon, etc.)

sea salt or plain salt

Directions:

Start by rinsing the quinoa under running water.

Then, add all the Ingredients: in a slow cooker and cover with a lid. Cook the mixture for 8 hours on low.

Serve hot with toppings of your choice.

Nutrition Info: Calories: 310, Total Fat: 16.8g, Saturated Fat: 13, Cholesterol: 0 mg, Sodium: 11 mg, Total Carbohydrate: 39 g, Dietary Fiber: 4.3 g, Total Sugars: 6.3 g, Protein: 7.4 g, Vitamin D: 0 mcg, Calcium: 30 mg, Iron: 3 mg, Potassium: 400 mg

Egg, Feta, Spinach, And Artichoke Freezer Breakfast Burritos

Servings: 6

Cooking Time: 5 Minutes

Ingredients:

8 large eggs

½ teaspoon dried Italian herbs

½ teaspoon garlic powder

½ teaspoon onion powder

3 teaspoons olive oil, divided

10 ounces baby spinach leaves

½ cup crumbled feta cheese

1 (14-ounce) can quartered artichoke hearts, super-tough leaves removed

6 (8- or 9-inch) whole-wheat tortillas

6 tablespoons prepared hummus or homemade hummus

Directions:

Beat the eggs and whisk in the Italian herbs, garlic powder, and onion powder.

Heat 1 teaspoon of oil in a 1inch skillet. When the oil is shimmering, add the spinach and sauté for 2 to 3 minutes, until the spinach is wilted. Remove the spinach from the pan.

In the same pan, heat the remaining 2 teaspoons of oil. When the oil is hot, add the eggs. When the eggs start to set, stir to scramble. Cook for about minutes, then add the cooked spinach, feta, and artichoke hearts. Cool the mixture and pour off any liquid if it accumulates.

Place 1 tortilla on a cutting board. Spread 1 tablespoon of hummus down the middle of the tortilla. Place ¾ cup of the egg filling on top of the hummus. Fold the bottom end and sides over the filling and tightly roll up. Repeat for the remaining 5 tortillas.

Wrap each burrito in foil and place in a resealable plastic bag.

STORAGE: Store sealed bags in the freezer for up to 3 months. To reheat burritos, unwrap and remove the foil. Cover the burrito with a damp paper towel, place on a microwaveable plate, and microwave on high until the center of the burrito is hot, about 2 minutes.

Nutrition Info: calories: 359; Total fat: 18g; Saturated fat: 6g; Sodium: 800mg; Carbohydrates: 32g; Fiber: 6g; Protein: 18g

Low Carb Waffles

Servings: 2

Cooking Time: 10 Minutes

Ingredients:

4 egg whites

2 whole eggs

½ teaspoon baking powder

4 tablespoons milk

4 tablespoons coconut flour

sugar or sweetener to taste

Directions:

Whip the egg whites to a stiff peak.

When the stiff peaks are attained, add the coconut flour, milk, baking powder, and the whole egg; mix.

Start heating your waffle iron to the required temperature. Grease it and pour in the batter. Cook until brown.

Serve warm and top with your choice of fruit or other toppings.

Nutrition Info: Calories: 234, Total Fat: 9.1g, Saturated Fat: 7, Cholesterol: 166 mg, Sodium: 204 mg, Total Carbohydrate: 18.9 g, Dietary Fiber: 10 g, Total Sugars: 4.2 g, Protein: 17.7 g, Vitamin D: 16 mcg, Calcium: 118 mg, Iron: 1 mg, Potassium: 310 mg

Potato Breakfast Hash

Servings: 2
Cooking Time: 10 Minutes

Ingredients:
1 sweet potato, diced
1 cup bell pepper, chopped
1 tsp cumin
1 tbsp olive oil
1 potato, diced
1/2 tsp pepper
1 tsp paprika
1/2 tsp garlic, minced
1/4 cup vegetable stock
1/2 tsp salt

Directions:
Add all ingredients into the instant pot and stir well.
Seal pot with lid and cook on high for 10 minutes.
Once done, release pressure using quick release. Remove lid. Stir and serve.

Nutrition Info: Calories: 206;Fat: 7.7 g; Carbohydrates: 32.9 g; Sugar: 7.6 g; Protein: 4 g; Cholesterol: 0 mg

Farro Porridge With Blackberry Compote

Servings: 4

Cooking Time: 30 Minutes

Ingredients:

1¼ cups uncooked semi-pearled farro

5 cups unsweetened vanilla almond milk

1 tablespoon pure maple syrup

1 (10-ounce) package frozen blackberries (2 cups)

2 teaspoons pure maple syrup

2 teaspoons balsamic vinegar

Directions:

TO MAKE THE FARRO.

Place the farro, almond milk, and maple syrup in a saucepan. Bring the liquid to a boil, then turn the heat down to low and simmer until the farro is tender and has absorbed much of the liquid, about 30 minutes. It should still look somewhat liquidy and will continue to absorb liquid as it cools.

Scoop ¾ cup of farro into each of 4 containers.

TO MAKE THE BLACKBERRY COMPOTE.

While the farro is cooking, place the frozen blackberries, maple syrup, and balsamic vinegar in a separate saucepan on medium-low heat. Cook for 12 to 1minutes, until the blackberry juices have thickened. Cool.

Spoon ¼ cup of the blackberry compote into each of the 4 farro containers.

STORAGE: Store covered containers in the refrigerator for up to 5 days.

Nutrition Info: Total calories: 334; Total fat: 5g; Saturated fat: 0g; Sodium: 227mg; Carbohydrates: 64g; Fiber: 11g; Protein: 11

Bulgur Fruit Breakfast Bowl

Servings: 6
Cooking Time: 15 Minutes

Ingredients:

2 cups 2% milk

½ teaspoon ground cinnamon

1 ½ cups bulgur

½ cup almonds, chopped

½ cup mint, chopped (fresh is preferred)

8 dried and chopped figs

1 cup water

2 cups frozen sweet cherries - you can also substitute in blueberries or blackberries

Directions:

Turn your stovetop to medium heat and combine the bulger, water, milk, and cinnamon. Lightly stir as the ingredients come to a boil.

Cover your mixture and turn the stove range temperature down to medium-low heat. Let the mixture simmer for 8 to 11 minutes. It is done simmering when about half of the liquid has been absorbed

Without removing the pan, turn off the range top heat and add the frozen cherries, almonds, and figs. Lightly stir and then cover for one minute so the cherries can thaw, and the mixture can combine.

Remove the cover and add in the mint before scooping your breakfast into a bowl.

Nutrition Info: calories: 301, fats: 6 grams, carbohydrates: grams, protein: 9 grams.

Acorn Squash Eggs

Servings: 5

Cooking Time: 30 Minutes

Ingredients:

2 acorn squash

4 eggs

2 tablespoons extra virgin olive oil

salt

pepper

5-6 dates, pitted

8 walnut halves

bunch fresh parsley

Directions:

Preheat oven to 375 degrees F.

Cut the squashes crosswise into ¾-inch thick slices; remove seeds.

Prepare slices with holes.

Line a baking sheet with parchment paper and place the slices on it.

Season with salt and pepper and bake for 20 minutes.

Chop up walnuts and dates.

Remove the baking dish from the oven and drizzle the slices with olive oil.

Crack an egg into the center of the slices (into the hole you made) and season with salt and pepper.

Sprinkle walnuts on top and put back in the oven for 10 minutes. Add maple syrup.

Enjoy!

Nutrition Info: Calories: 198, Total Fat: 9.5g, Saturated Fat: 2, Cholesterol: 131 mg, Sodium: 97 mg, Total Carbohydrate: 25.7 g, Dietary Fiber: 3.9 g, Total Sugars: 5.7 g, Protein: 6.6 g, Vitamin D: mcg, Calcium: 107 mg, Iron: 3 mg, Potassium: 811 mg

Green Smoothie

Servings: 2
Cooking Time: 12 Minutes

Ingredients:
4 cups spinach
20 almonds, raw
2 cups milk
2 scoops whey protein
sweetener of your choice and to taste

Directions:
Start by blending spinach, almond, and milk in a blender.
Blend until the puree is formed.
Add the rest of the Ingredients: and blend well.
Pour into glasses and serve.
Enjoy.

Nutrition Info: Calories: 325, Total Fat: 13.1 g, Saturated Fat: 4.4 g, Cholesterol: 85 mg, Sodium: 218 mg, Total Carbohydrate: 20.4 g, Dietary Fiber: 2.8 g, Total Sugars: 12.7 g, Protein: 34.4 g, Vitamin D: 1 mcg, Calcium: 482 mg, Iron: 3 mg, Potassium: 738 mg .

Thick Pomegranate Cherry Smoothie

Servings: 4

Cooking Time: 5 Minutes

Ingredients:

16 ounces frozen dark cherries

¾ cup pomegranate juice

1 teaspoon vanilla extract

6 ice cubes

½ cup pomegranate seeds

1 ½ cups Greek yogurt, plain

⅓ cup milk

¾ teaspoon ground cinnamon

½ cup pistachios, chopped

Directions:

Add the ice cubes, cherries, pomegranate juice, yogurt, vanilla, milk, and cinnamon into a blender. Mix until the ingredients are smooth. It is thicker than your average smoothie.

Instead of a cup, divide the smoothie into four bowls.

Sprinkle chopped pistachios and pomegranate seeds on top of the smoothie.

Serve and enjoy!

Nutrition Info: calories: 212, fats: 7 grams, carbohydrates: 3grams, protein: 4 grams.

Honey Nut Granola

Servings: 6

Cooking Time: 30 Minutes

Ingredients:

¼ cup honey

2 ½ cups rolled oats

¼ teaspoon sea salt

2 tablespoons ground flaxseed

2 teaspoons vanilla extract

⅓ cup chopped almonds

½ teaspoon ground cinnamon

¼ cup olive oil

½ cup dried apricots, chopped

Directions:

Set the temperature of your oven to 325 degrees Fahrenheit and line a baking pan with a piece of parchment paper. While you can grease the pan, it is easier to use parchment paper when you're cutting the granola.

Turn a burner on your stovetop to medium heat and add the salt, chopped almonds, cinnamon, and oats. Cook the mixture for 5 to 6 minutes while stirring occasionally.

Using a microwavable-safe dish, mix the flaxseed, apricots, oil, and honey. Set the mixture in your microwave and the timer for

1 minute. If the mixture does not bubble within the minute, continue for another minute or until the mixture bubbles.

Mix the vanilla into the flaxseed mixture and then pour this mixture over the almond and oats mixture. Combine the ingredients thoroughly.

Remove the skillet from heat and pour onto the parchment paper. Spread the mixture as evenly as possible with a spatula or another sheet of parchment paper and your hand.

Set the pan into the oven and turn your timer to 15 minutes. However, you want to watch the granola closely as once it starts to brown, you'll need to remove it from heat.

Set the granola aside to cool thoroughly. If you used parchment paper, you can take the granola out of the pan by holding the paper and setting it on your counter. It will cool faster so you can eat it faster! Once this waiting is done, cut or break apart the granola into small pieces and enjoy!

Nutrition Info: calories: 337, fats: 17 grams, carbohydrates: 42 grams, protein: 7 grams.

Quinoa Granola

Servings: 2

Cooking Time: 25 Minutes

Ingredients:

1 cup Old-Fashioned rolled oats, or gluten-free

1/2 cup uncooked white quinoa

2 cups raw almonds, roughly chopped

1 Tbsp coconut sugar or sub organic brown sugar, muscovado, or organic cane sugar

1 pinch sea salt

3 1/2 tbsp coconut oil

1/4 cup maple syrup or agave nectar

Directions:

Preheat oven to 340 degrees F

In a large mixing bowl, add the quinoa, almonds, oats, coconut sugar, and salt, stir to combine

To a small saucepan, add the maple syrup and coconut oil, warm over medium heat for 2-minutes, whisking frequently until completely mixed and combined

Immediately pour over the dry ingredients, stir to combine and thoroughly all oats and nuts

Arrange on a large baking sheet, spread into an even layer

Bake for 20 minutes

Then remove from oven, stir and toss the granola - make sure to turn the pan around so the other end goes into the oven first and bakes
evenly

Bake for 5-10 minutes more - watch carefully so it doesn't burn and it's golden brown and very fragrant

Allow to cool completely, then store in a container for up to 7 days

Nutrition Info: Calories:332; Total Carbohydrates: 30g; Total Fat: 20g; Protein: 9g

Greek Yogurt With Fresh Berries, Honey And Nuts

Servings: 1

Cooking Time: 5 Minutes

Ingredients:

6 oz. nonfat plain Greek yogurt

1/2 cup fresh berries of your choice

1 tbsp .25 oz crushed walnuts

1 tbsp honey

Directions:

In a jar with a lid, add the yogurt

Top with berries and a drizzle of honey

Top with the lid and store in the fridge for 2-days

To Serve: Add the granola or nuts, enjoy

Nutrition Info: Calories:2;Carbs: 35g;Total Fat: 4g;Protein: 19g

www.ingramcontent.com/pod-product-compliance
Lightning Source LLC
Chambersburg PA
CBHW070730030426
42336CB00013B/1931